T0144639

BASIC HEALTH
PUBLICATIONS
USER'S GUIDE

TO NATURAL REMEDIES FOR DEPRESSION

*Learn about Safe and
Natural Treatments to
Uplift Your Mood
and Conquer
Depression.*

LINDA KNITTEL, M.A.

JACK CHALLEM Series Editor

The information contained in this book is based upon the research and personal and professional experiences of the author. It is not intended as a substitute for consulting with your physician or other healthcare provider. Any attempt to diagnose and treat an illness should be done under the direction of a healthcare professional.

The publisher does not advocate the use of any particular healthcare protocol but believes the information in this book should be available to the public. The publisher and author are not responsible for any adverse effects or consequences resulting from the use of the suggestions, preparations, or procedures discussed in this book. Should the reader have any questions concerning the appropriateness of any procedures or preparations mentioned, the author and the publisher strongly suggest consulting a professional healthcare advisor.

Series Editor: Jack Challem
Editor: Rowan Jacobson
Typesetter: Gary A. Rosenberg
Series Cover Designer: Mike Stromberg

Basic Health Publications User's Guides are published by Basic Health Publications, Inc.

CONTENTS

INTRODUCTION

Do you awake each morning feeling hope-less, irritable, and just plain sad? If so, there are two important things you should know: first, you *can* feel better, and second, you are not alone.

According to the American Medical Associa-tion, one in ten adult Americans will suffer from depression in any given year. That's more than 17 million people looking for a way to ease their sadness, anxiety, and fatigue—a number that has made the pharmaceutical companies quite jolly. But natural treatments for depression are begin-ning to give the big drugs a run for their money. More and more people are discovering that herbs, vitamins, minerals, and lifestyle changes are powerful enough to lift depression and its symptoms without the unwanted side effects that often accompany drugs. In other words, most natural approaches to depression have safety records that blow their pharmaceutical counter-parts out of the water.

If you think you or someone you know is suf-fering from depression, then read on, for this book will explain how to overcome depression using all-natural treatments that will not only lift your mood but also improve your overall health and well-being.

There is no denying that traditional approach-es to treating depression—such as the daily use of antidepressant drugs—have helped numerous people, but these substances often cause serious side effects and can be fairly addictive. In contrast, natural treatments such as diet, herbs, vitamins, and other nutrients have shown to be equally or more effective at elevating mood and have demonstrated few side effects.

In this *User's Guide to Natural Treatments for Depression,* you will learn that depression is often brought on by a combination of external influences and chemical imbalances in the brain. When these chemicals are returned to normal levels—via herbs, light therapy, diet, exercise, or supplements—one naturally feels better. Each chapter of this book is designed to address a single natural approach to treating depression and its symptoms, so you can understand the science behind each treatment and learn the proper methods and doses for its use.

Although one of the strongest appeals of these natural approaches is that they can be used without a prescription, it is important to seek the guidance of a physician or other health practitioner when beginning any treatment program. Additionally, since there are many types of mood disorders, it is recommended that you seek professional help in determining the exact nature of your condition, as well as your individual health concerns. But remember, the power to overcome your depression is in your hands. If you believe you can get well, and are willing to do a little research and make a few healthy lifestyle changes, then relief is just around the corner.

CHAPTER 1

WHAT IS DEPRESSION?

Each day, millions of people struggle with feelings of worthlessness, sadness, and despair. Although external factors such as work, family, and finances can contribute to one's melancholy, scientific research shows that most mood disorders—including depression—are also linked to levels of certain brain chemicals. When these chemicals are not present in sufficient quantities, or are not able to function properly, mood disturbances arise. The good news is that in most cases you can balance these chemicals by natural means, without having to resort to prescription antidepressants.

How Does Depression Differ from Just Being Sad?

Certainly everybody feels sad from time to time, but unlike occasional sadness, depression is characterized by persistent blue moods. Not only do these moods tend to interfere with major life activities such as work, family, or school, but they also have a strong negative effect on an individual's self-esteem. Someone who is depressed often feels exhausted, hopeless, and disinterested in life in general.

Like most conditions, there are varying degrees of depressive states. Mild depression describes a condition in which one suffers from some symptoms, but is able to carry out daily responsibilities. Moderate depression occurs when symptoms prevent one from doing what needs to be done, whereas major depression exists when one's sadness completely overwhelms the ability to cope with everyday life.

The Symptoms of Depression

1. Prolonged sadness
2. Excessive crying
3. Fatigue or difficulty sleeping
4. Loss of sex drive
5. Changes in eating patterns
6. Anxiety
7. Hopelessness
8. Irritability
9. Changes in weight
10. Suicidal thoughts

As mentioned in the Introduction, at least 17 million American adults—1 in 10—suffer from depression in any given year. Furthermore, women are twice as likely to become depressed as men. While depression is found in all age groups, it is most common in middle-aged adults.

There are several theories as to why more women are treated for depression than men. Possibly, this is due to the high stress levels women face in their conflicting roles at work and home. The constant hormonal changes that women experience are another factor. Then again, women may simply be more likely to seek help than men, thus, they appear to have higher rates of depression. The truth undoubtedly lies in a combination of all three explanations.

It also appears that some forms of depression do run in families. This is especially common of bipolar depression.

Types of Depression

There are many different levels of mood disorders, each with its own set of characteristics and symptoms. The most common forms are major depression and bipolar depression. Some additional forms of depression include cyclothymia, dysthymia, seasonal affective disorder, and postpartum depression.

Bipolar Depression

A condition, sometimes called manic-depressive illness, characterized by dramatic oscillations between feelings of depression and euphoria.

Cyclothymia is a mild form of bipolar depression that usually develops in early adult life and is characterized by frequent periods of both depression and mild elation. Dysthymia, on the other hand, is a condition of mild, constant depression that usually lasts for more than two years. Often dysthymia begins early in life and is marked by feelings of hopelessness, low self-esteem, and irritability. Seasonal affective disorder (SAD) is a type of depression that occurs during specific times of the year when light patterns are altered. Most often, individuals suffering from SAD feel depressed during the gray winter months and happy during the summer. Symptoms include fatigue, increase in appetite, difficulty concentrating, sadness, and anxiety. Postpartum depression describes a severe, prolonged period of sadness in women following the birth of a child.

Childbirth and Depression

As mentioned above, depression appears to be twice as common in women as it is in men, with its greatest incidence during the primary reproductive years—ages twenty-five to forty-five. The link between reproductive status and depressive illness appears as depression during the premenstrual phase, the perimenopausal period, and the immediate postpartum period.

Despite the fact that postpartum depression has recently made a name for itself in the popular press, this condition remains a frequently overlooked illness—despite the potentially horrific consequences. Because of the major physical, psychological, and social changes that accompany childbirth, it is certainly a major risk factor in the development of mental illness. Of the approximately four million births occurring annually in this country, nearly 40 percent involve some form of a postpartum mood disorder.

In a trial published in *Psychological Medicine*, researchers reviewed the outcomes of more than 35,000 deliveries. Through ninety-day interval screenings over a two-year period preceding and following each delivery, the team found a sevenfold increase in the risk of psychiatric hospitalization in the first three months after delivery. Researchers also found the risk of psychosis to be twenty-two times higher than the prepregnancy rate.

What Is Postpartum Depression?

Generally, the realm of postpartum mood disorders is divided into three distinct categories. At one end of the spectrum is the "baby blues," a common phenomenon categorized by low mood, irritability, anxiety, crying, insomnia, and changes in appetite. Typically, these symptoms occur in the first few days after delivery. A supportive environment and the settling down of hormones usually resolves such symptoms.

Postpartum Depression
A severe, prolonged period of sadness in women following the birth of their child.

At the other end of the spectrum is the infrequently occurring puerperal psychosis, a condition that usually emerges within the first four weeks postpartum, but which can appear up to ninety days after delivery. Women suffering from this condition experience desires to hurt themselves or their babies. In the middle of these two extremes is postpartum depression, a condition believed to involve 10 to 15 percent of all deliveries. For the majority of patients who suffer from this illness, symptoms last more than six months. If untreated, an estimated 25 percent of these women will still be depressed a year later.

There is no reason to believe that postpartum depression responds differently to treatment than other types of mood disorders. However, due to the delicate nature of infants' safety, early identification and treatment of the condition are essential. If you suspect that you or someone you love is suffering from this condition, seek the advice of a health care practitioner right away.

Natural treatment options are especially preferable while breastfeeding. Light therapy can be a great option (see Chapter 9), and a number of the nutrients and herbs mentioned in this book can be used safely with the help of a knowledgeable physician.

What Causes Depression?

Although the exact causes of depression are not fully understood, it is clear that three elements—genetics, biology, and environment—contribute to its development. Genetic causes include an inherited susceptibility to depression, biological causes involve fluctuations in hormones in the body or secretions in the brain, and environmental reasons include seasons and stressful or sad emotional situations. Most often, depressive illness is brought on by an interaction of two or more of these causes.

In her pioneering book *The Way Up from Down*, Priscilla Slagle, M.D., outlines what is called the "brain amine theory of depression." This theory is based on the knowledge that certain chemicals—called neurotransmitters—are released by nerve endings in the brain. These chemicals move from one cell to another, creating either positive "rewarding" thoughts or negative "punishing" ones. Once these chemicals have transmitted their message, they are broken down by special chemicals such as monoamine oxidase. This causes a small amount of the neurotransmitters' building blocks (amines) to be excreted in the urine, while the majority (85 percent) are reabsorbed by the cell that released them. This process is called reuptake.

It has been discovered that the cells of depressed individuals are often either unable to properly receive neurotransmitters or are unable to properly perform reuptake. In addition, depressed people often have too little of the amines needed to create these neurotransmitters. If the necessary amines (serotonin and norepinephrine) are not present in the right quantities, depression may result. Studies seem to indicate that these neurotransmitter malfunctions are genetically inherited.

Neurotransmitters
Chemicals used to carry messages throughout the brain's network of cells.

Conventional Treatments for Depression

Although many of today's professionals acknowledge the role nutrition and psychotherapy can play in the management of depression, the most common treatment is a program of antidepressant drugs. These drugs are used to lift an individual's mood by altering the levels of chemicals in the brain.

The most commonly prescribed antidepressant drugs fall into three different categories, depending on how they work in the body. Selective serotonin reuptake inhibitors (SSRIs), such as

Prozac, prevent cells from performing reuptake, thus boosting serotonin levels in the brain. Tricyclic antidepressants (TCAs), like Tofranil, enhance the potency of neurotransmitters in the brain. And monoamine oxidase inhibitors (MAOIs), such as Parnate, prevent the substance monoamine oxidase from breaking down sero-

Serotonin
One of the brain's principal neurotransmitters, responsible for regulating mood.

tonin, dopamine, and norepinephrine, thus increasing their supply and improving mood.

Each specific antidepressant drug has its own set of side effects, but in general they include elevated blood pressure, rapid heartbeat, constipation, dry mouth, blurred vision, skin rashes, weight gain, hallucinations, anxiety, nightmares, insomnia, numbness, tingling, ringing in the ears, loss of coordination, and seizures. If you are considering taking antidepressant medication, be sure to educate yourself on the potential side effects.

Although antidepressant drugs have been successful in treating numerous people, as many as 30 percent of depressed individuals do not respond to these drugs. In addition, these medications can take up to six weeks to become effective, and a lapse in use can often bring about a relapse in symptoms.

Alternatives to Antidepressant Drugs

In the past decade, numerous scientific studies have confirmed what herbalists and nutritionists have known for centuries, that certain naturally occurring substances can simulate the same processes in the brain as antidepressant drugs. Furthermore, approaches using light therapy, nutrition, and lifestyle modification can drastically improve the mood of depressed individuals. All of these approaches will be discussed in detail in subsequent chapters.

CHAPTER 2

RULING OUT
MEDICAL CAUSES

The daunting truth is that there are at least one hundred physical conditions whose symptoms look strikingly like those of mild to moderate depression. If left untreated, these conditions can not only keep you depressed, but can also wreak havoc on your physical health. Therefore, the best first step to treating any case of depression is a full physical exam. Once it has been determined that your poor emotional state is not the result of a hidden physical problem, steps can be taken to improve your mood naturally. A handful of these conditions discussed below, including candida, hypothyroidism, and hormonal imbalances, are quite common and can exist undetected for long periods of time. If any of these conditions seem in line with your symptoms, be sure to seek the opinion of a knowledgeable physician.

What Is Candida?

It may not be a pleasant thought, but several types of harmless yeast and fungi live in different areas of our bodies at any given time. And the truth is, when the fungus responsible for candida—*Candida albicans*—exists in normal amounts in the mouth area, gastrointestinal tract, or vagina, there is no cause for alarm. But if this yeast is allowed to grow out of control, it begins to damage the delicate lining of the intestines, permitting toxins, undigested protein particles, and

Candida
An infection caused by an overgrowth of yeast in the body.

the yeast itself to pass directly into the blood stream. Believing these substances to be antigens or foreign invaders, the body then initiates an antibody reaction, resulting in inflammation, fatigue, bloating, allergies, headaches and depression.

Sadly, the symptoms of candida are becoming more widespread now that excessive antibiotic use, heavily refined diets, abundant environmental toxins, and the use of birth control and hormone replacement pills are part of many people's everyday lives. That is because these so-called luxuries of our modern lifestyle place strain on the immune system, and disrupt the natural defense systems that keep yeast levels in check. Fortunately, a few not-so-modern treatments, such as herbs, supplements, and fresh whole foods, can restore balance to your delicate inner ecology and keep candida at bay.

Symptoms of Candida

Occasionally, blood tests will reveal a candida overgrowth, but generally, the condition must be diagnosed based on a patient's health history and current clinical picture. A history of chronic antibiotic use, chronic vaginal yeast infections, oral birth control use, a heavily refined diet, and use of hormone replacement therapy (HRT) are frequent precursors to candida. The symptoms of candida can be varied, but the most common include depression, chronic fatigue, constipation and/or diarrhea, bloating, acne, headaches, allergies, and sugar cravings.

Treating Candida with Diet

The first step in ridding the body of candida is to deprive the yeast of its favorite food: sugar. In fact, in a study published in the *Journal of Repro-*

ductive Medicine, out of 49 women suffering from candida-related vaginal infections, 90 percent of those who reduced their intake of sugar drastically reduced the incidence and severity of such infections over the next year. Therefore, it is best to avoid all refined sugar, including packaged foods that contain sugar, and to eliminate or drastically reduce your consumption of honey, maple syrup, fruit, fruit juice, and simple carbohydrates such as pasta, white rice, white bread, and potatoes.

Dairy products should also be avoided, because the lactose they contain has been shown to promote candida growth. Likewise, you should steer clear of foods that contain yeast or mold such as mushrooms, alcohol, cheeses, melons, dried fruit, and fermented products like soy sauce and vinegar.

What should you eat to promote a healthy gut? The bulk of the diet should be fiber-rich, low-carbohydrate vegetables. Modest amounts of fish, poultry, and lean meat can also be eaten along with unprocessed oils, nuts, seeds, and plenty of purified water. Although practitioners will differ on exactly which foods should be avoided and which can be eaten safely, most agree that switching to a low-carbohydrate, sugar-free diet is the most important step in the fight against candida.

Supplements That Treat Candida

Along with dietary changes, a number of herbs and supplements can help eliminate yeast and promote a healthy digestive tract. For example, studies have shown that the antibiotic and antimicrobial properties in herbs such as garlic (*Allium sativum*), barberry (*Berberis vulgaris*), oregano (*Oreganium vulgare*), Oregon grape (*Berberis aquifolium*) and goldenseal (*Hydrastis canaden-*

sis), as well as caprylic acid, can inhibit the growth of yeast.

Boosting the amount of probiotics—good bacteria—that exists in your body can also keep the digestive tract in balance. To do so, supplement with strains of flora such as *Lactobacillus acidophilus, Bifidobacterium bifidum,* and *Lactobacillus bulgaricus,* as well as fructo-oligosaccharides (FOS)—a soluble fiber on which these bacteria thrive.

Probiotics
Friendly bacteria that keep the digestive tract working smoothly.

A host of other supplements have shown promise in treating the symptoms of candida. For instance, antioxidants like vitamins C and E, and essential fatty acids such as flaxseed, can help protect intestinal cell membranes, while the amino acid L-glutamine is known to help repair damage to the gut wall. As with any herb or supplement regimen, it is important to work with a knowledgeable health practitioner to determine a protocol and dosages that will be safe and effective for you.

Although over-the-counter anti-yeast medications do exist, they generally provide only temporary relief since they do not address the underlying reasons why a candida overgrowth has occurred. Therefore, only a comprehensive approach, including dietary changes and natural supplements, will rid your body of yeast overgrowth and prevent it from ever coming back.

What Is Hypothyroidism?

An estimated 11 million Americans—9 million of which are women—suffer from an underactive thyroid. Given that the thyroid gland is responsible for regulating countless functions in the body, including metabolism, it makes sense that the underproduction of thyroid hormones—known as hypothyroidism—would lead to a whole host of symptoms ranging from weight gain and fatigue to infertility and depression.

The small, butterfly-shaped thyroid gland sits at the base of the throat, where it excretes hormones, mainly thyroxine (known as T4) and triiodothyronine (known as T3). The foremost job of these hormones is to help cells convert

Hypothyroidism
A debilitating condition caused by an underproduction of thyroid hormones.

calories and oxygen into energy. This process can be interrupted by a variety of factors, including treatment for other thyroid conditions, iodine deficiency, pregnancy, and congenital abnormalities. But most often, hypothyroidism is due to an autoimmune condition known as Hashimoto's thyroiditis, in which antibodies attack the thyroid and render it inactive.

Risk Factors for Hypothyroidism

"Women are much more prone to autoimmune diseases, which is one of the reasons why we see more hypothyroidism in women," says M. Sara Rosenthal, author of *The Hypothyroid Sourcebook.* Pregnancy, menopause, and a greater life expectancy also contribute to the higher rates of this condition in women. There also seems to be a relationship between progesterone deficiency and hypothyroidism. When progesterone receptors malfunction due to factors such as stress or low blood sugar, the thyroid does not work right either.

Since most PMS symptoms are due to a deficiency in progesterone, women who are suffering from severe PMS should be sure to have their thyroid checked. Many experts believe everyone should have their thyroid tested yearly. The test is cheap, and often the condition will go undiagnosed for years otherwise. However, the American Thyroid Association promotes screening only for those thirty-five and older, while the American College of Physicians/American Society of Internal Medicine advocates screening for women age fifty and up.

Symptoms of Hypothyroidism

Given that hypothyroidism is not usually preventable, one's best defense is to catch it early by recognizing the signs. If you suffer from a number of the following symptoms, talk to your practitioner about thyroid testing: depression, weight gain, slow healing, shortness of breath, cold sensations, fatigue, constipation, brittle nails and hair, difficulty concentrating, headaches, or irregular periods.

Frequently, a practitioner will first ask a potentially hypothyroidal patient to keep track of his or her basal body temperature for a few days to see if it is running low. If it clocks in under 97.6 degrees several mornings in a row, she will prescribe a TSH test, which measures the level of thyroid stimulating hormone in the blood. Since lab tests are not an exact science, it is always best to ask for further testing if you are not satisfied with the results.

Treating Hypothyroidism

Even the *British Medical Journal* recently acknowledged that TSH test results can be ambiguous and confusing, suggesting that the best way to determine who should receive thyroid treatment is not by a set number, but by how a patient feels. Even if your lab readings and your doctor are telling you that you are fine, you may be helped by hormone replacement. A few well-controlled clinical trials have confirmed this to be true, showing that even individuals suffering from mild hypothyroidism benefit from treatment. And since thyroid dysfunction generally worsens over time, early treatment can prevent more serious health problems.

Most holistic practitioners prescribe desiccated thyroid sourced from the glands of pigs, because it contains both T4 and T3. In theory, the body will produce T3 from T4. For this reason, most conventional practitioners have considered supplementation with synthetic T4 (levothyroxine) a safe and adequate means of treatment. However, recent research published in the *New England Journal of Medicine* suggests that there are individuals who may benefit from adding synthetic T3 to their conventional medication regimen. The bottom line? There is no blanket medication recipe for everyone, so it is important to work with a skilled practitioner when treating this condition.

What Is PMS?

Although estimates vary, at least 60 percent of American women suffer from debilitating symptoms such as depression, mood swings, and fatigue during the days prior to menstruation. The large majority of these symptoms—collectively known as premenstrual syndrome (PMS)—are the result of hormonal imbalances.

PMS
Hormone-related symptoms such as depression, bloating, mood swings, and fatigue that occur prior to menstruation.

By and large, PMS symptoms can be controlled. Women with PMS symptoms generally have elevated estrogen levels in relation to progesterone. Factors such as stress, environmental toxins (such as pesticides), and a diet high in estrogenic and refined foods can greatly contribute to this condition. By eliminating these factors—including foods such as commercial meat and dairy products, sugar, caffeine, and alcohol—a woman can markedly ease her monthly symptoms.

How do I Know if I Have PMS?

Although the majority of women experience some PMS symptoms, up to 10 percent of menstruating women are actually incapacitated by these hormone-related conditions. Generally, if you suffer from five or more PMS symptoms, and experience a significant monthly mood change that affects your work, relationships, or life in general, then you should absolutely seek help. In addition to considering the following symptoms, checking in with friends and family can often shed light on how drastically your hormones affect you each month.

The most common PMS symptoms include acne, anxiety, bloating, breast tenderness, clumsiness, cramps, crying spells, depression, dizziness, headaches, insomnia, intestinal disturbances, lower back pain, mood swings, sugar cravings, and weight gain.

Vegetarian Diet Eases PMS

Although what a woman does *not* eat may be one of the most effective ways of preventing PMS, there are also a number of desirable foods that actually work to help keep estrogen levels low. For example, a recent study in *Obstetrics and Gynecology* found that consuming a low-fat vegetarian diet—full of vegetables, fruits, legumes, and whole grains—significantly reduced PMS symptoms. A low-fat diet is believed to help increase sex hormone binding globulin in the blood, which is what keeps our hormones from floating around and being overactive. In addition, a vegetarian diet is high in the fiber needed to bind up estrogen in the intestinal tract and shuttle it out of the body.

One more way eating like a vegetarian can promote healthy estrogen levels is through the use of soy protein. Soy is a plant compound that binds to estrogen receptors in the body and exerts one of two effects. When estrogen levels are low, soy foods can exert a weak estrogenic effect. When there is too much estrogen—as is the case with PMS—the isoflavones in soy bind to estrogen receptors and block the body's own estrogen from causing painful symptoms.

Nutrients for PMS Relief

Certain nutrient-rich foods, including those packed with omega-3 fatty acids, magnesium, and calcium, may also help relieve the symptoms of PMS. According to a recent study published in the *American Journal of Obstetrics and Gynecology,* women who took 1,200 mg of calcium a day for three months cut their food cravings, mood swings, and water retention in half. To get more calcium in your diet, reach for broccoli, spinach, kale, and figs.

Studies of magnesium's effect on PMS also look promising. A double-blind placebo-controlled trial revealed that after two months of supplementation with 200 mg of magnesium, symptoms such as weight gain, swelling, breast tenderness, and abdominal bloating were significantly reduced. Magnesium is crucial for the formation of mood-regulating neurotransmitters. A few good food sources of magnesium include lima beans, kale, nuts, and pumpkinseeds.

Omega-3-rich foods can also help to prevent PMS by promoting the production of the good prostaglandins, which fight inflammation. Salmon and flaxseeds are two excellent sources.

CHAPTER 3

ST. JOHN'S WORT

Numerous scientific studies have now proven what traditional herbalists have known for ages: that the herb St. John's wort does indeed elevate mood. In fact, cutting-edge scientific studies have demonstrated that St. John's wort is often more effective than antidepressant drugs at treating mild to moderate depression. Furthermore, this herb can be taken with few, if any, side effects. This chapter will explain what St. John's wort is, how it works in the body, and how to use it properly.

What Is St. John's Wort?

St. John's wort, or *Hypericum perforatum,* is an abundant yellow-flowered plant whose medicinal properties have been valued for thousands of years. Once regarded as simply an unruly weed that grows all over sun-exposed slopes in Europe, Asia, and the United States, St. John's wort's benefits have been recently rediscovered.

Botanists believe that St. John's wort evolved hundreds of millions of years before humans. The first written accounts of its use are found in ancient Greek and Roman texts, which document its effectiveness in the treatment of burns, infections, and snake bites, and as protection from evil spirits. St. John's wort's uses were passed down through generations of early Europeans, and its healing properties were also well utilized by Native Americans.

Not until the end of the nineteenth century,

when herbal medicine was forced underground, did St. John's wort became less prominent. Aside from places like Germany, where herbal medicine has always reigned supreme, St. John's wort was overlooked for decades.

Renewed Interest in St. John's Wort

We now have sound, scientific evidence that St. John's wort can relieve a number of chronic conditions. In 1996, the *British Medical Journal* published an overview of twenty-three clinical trials to determine St. John's wort's effectiveness in relieving depression. The study looked at trials that had pinned St. John's wort against a placebo, as well as trials that had compared St. John's wort to standard antidepressants. It found that individuals suffering from mild to moderate depression fared better with St. John's wort (63.9 percent of patients improved) than with conventional antidepressants (58.5 percent). In addition, the number of patients who were forced to drop out of the study due to standard antidepressant side effects (3.0 percent) was much higher than with those taking St. John's wort (0.8 percent).

The Effects of St. John's Wort

Exactly how St. John's wort works and the makeup of its active components is still a mystery. However, because it produces the same sort of effects as the SSRIs such as Prozac, researchers believe that the herb, like those antidepressants, slows down the rate at which the brain reabsorbs serotonin, thus leaving more of the neurotransmitter available for reception. Some research demonstrates that St. John's wort may also alter concentrations of other neurotransmitters, as well as increase receptor-site sensitivity.

It appears that St. John's wort's active ingredients must build up in the body (usually 4–6 weeks) before bringing about their full effect. However, many users find some symptom relief—such as better sleep, decreased anxiety, and more energy—within the first week to ten days. After a few weeks, most people (70 percent) experience positive results such as an increase in mood and a stronger feeling of emotional balance.

Other Uses of St. John's Wort

Germany's Commission E—an organization similar to the American Food and Drug Administration—has approved St. John's wort's topical use for treating wounds, bruises, and burns, and its oral use for treating stomach and gastrointestinal conditions. Additional reports indicate that St. John's wort is effective in treating panic attacks, PMS, menopause, viral infections, and other chronic conditions. Clearly, all of its uses have not yet been determined.

Treating Depression with St. John's Wort

If you think you may be suffering from mild to moderate depression, St. John's wort holds great promise for you. However, be sure to first work with a health professional to determine the exact degree of your condition and to map out an appropriate treatment plan.

Since herbs such as St. John's wort contain numerous active ingredients, it is important to establish a standard by which each product must be measured. At one time, the active ingredient hypericin was thought to be the main mood-elevating component of St. John's wort, so many supplements are standardized using this component as a guide. When buying these St. John's wort products, look for a label that lists a 0.3 percent concentration of hypericin. That would mean that there are .09 mg of the ingredient in a 300 mg tablet.

Recent studies suggest that a separate ingredient—hyperforin—is the primary antidepressant compound in St. John's wort. When buying St. John's wort supplements standardized by this ingredient, look for a label that

Hyperforin
An active ingredient in St. John's wort that is generally used to standardize the herb. Look for a product with 3 percent hyperforin.

lists a 3 percent concentration of hyperforin, equivalent to 9 mg of the ingredient in a 300 mg tablet. In addition, look for products that are solely made from unopened buds, as they are the most potent, although those made from a combination of buds and opened flowers are quite powerful as well.

Forms of St. John's Wort

Tinctures of St. John's wort are believed to be the most powerful form, as the ingredients are the most well preserved. They are created by soaking the crushed herb in alcohol or glycerin, allowing the herb's oil to seep into the liquid, straining out the residue, and storing the liquid in a tinted bottle. St. John's wort also comes in tablets and capsules made from powdered, dried herb. These supplements vary in sizes and strengths, so it is important to make sure you are buying and taking the proper dosage.

Don't hesitate to call product companies and ask for proof that their particular St. John's wort product has been proven to work in controlled clinical trials. Extracts of such products usually carry a special research code and patent reference on the label.

How to Use St. John's Wort

It is often recommended to begin your program by taking 300 mg of St. John's wort and increasing the dose gradually until you reach 900 mg per day. Although research shows that the average successful dose is 300 mg three times daily, some people require less and some need more. Experiment to find a dose that works for you, especially if you are opting to use St. John's wort in tincture form. When using St. John's wort tincture, you may want to start with one dropperful per day and build up to two dropperfuls 2–3 times per day.

Although the active ingredients in St. John's wort are effective for more than twenty-four hours, it is best not to take your dose all at once. By breaking up the times you take your doses— such as at breakfast, lunch, and dinner—you will keep a steady concentration of the herb in the body and will prevent possible stomach upset.

Possible Side Effects of Taking St. John's Wort

Unlike standard antidepressants, which often cause bothersome side effects such as drowsiness, sleep disorders, and loss of concentration, St. John's wort has generally been shown to produce very few, and very mild, side effects.

In 1994, a research team performed a drug-monitoring study using 3,250 patients, which showed that only 2.4 percent of St. John's wort users experienced mild side effects such as gastrointestinal disturbances and anxiety. Most additional studies show similar or even lower rates of undesired effects.

Occasionally, St. John's wort will cause a heightened sensitivity to sunlight. Symptoms of photosensitivity include susceptibility to sunburn, skin rash, and pain or burning of the skin after sun exposure. If you are fair-skinned or have sensitive skin, limit sun exposure while taking St. John's wort.

If you experience any severe side effect such as dizziness or weakness while taking St. John's wort, you should discontinue use immediately.

St. John's Wort and Prescription Drugs

Recent studies suggest that St. John's wort may interact with certain medications such as birth control pills, blood thinners, the HIV drug indinavir, and organ transplant drugs, as well as various heart, asthma, and antiseizure medications. Therefore, individuals who have a medical condition, high blood pressure, are on medication, or are over sixty-five should absolutely consult a physician before taking St. John's wort. Furthermore, there has not yet been enough research on St. John's wort's effects on pregnant and breastfeeding women, or children under the age of twelve, to assure its safety for these individuals.

Although there have been no official long-term studies of St. John's wort use, it has been used safely and without ill effects for years. Hence, it appears the herb can be taken as long as necessary. As with any antidepressant, it may be wise to continue its use for a short while after the symptoms of depression subside. And when you do stop, it is a good idea to taper off gradually, monitoring your symptoms carefully, so as to avoid a relapse.

Using St. John's Wort with Other Antidepressants

No adverse reactions have been reported as the result of combining St. John's wort and MAO inhibitors or tricyclics. Nevertheless, because St. John's wort is a natural antidepressant rather than a synthetic one, and because it has far fewer side effects, you may want to consider switching if you currently take a synthetic antidepressant. A change of this kind should only be undertaken gradually, and with a doctor's supervision.

CHAPTER 4

S-ADENOSYL-L-METHIONINE (SAMe)

One of the newest antidepressant supplements to hit the market is the multipurpose compound S-adenosyl-L-methionine (SAMe). Although its name may sound synthetic, SAMe (pronounced *sammy*) is a naturally occurring compound produced in the body. SAMe's ability to donate one of its methyl groups makes it an integral part of many biochemical processes, including mood elevation, liver support, tissue formation, and so on. This chapter outlines how SAMe works in the body and what benefits SAMe supplementation may bring.

What Is SAMe?

SAMe is a natural substance formed by the combination of the amino acid L-methionine with ATP (adenosine triphosphate), the main energy molecule used in most bodily processes. Once formed, SAMe, or "active methionine," donates its activated S-methyl group for use in any of three different methylation processes (transmethylation, transsulfuration, and aminopropylation).

Methylation

A process, central to mood control, among other functions, in which a molecule donates one of its methyl groups to another substance in the body.

The process of methylation is critical to more than forty biochemical reactions in the body. At the most basic level, methylation has a direct impact on the health and replication of the body's building blocks, DNA. In addition, the process of methylation helps keep the liver healthy, helps generate proteins in the body, breaks down fats, and produces chemicals in the brain that control mood.

How SAMe Improves the Symptoms of Depression

Since SAMe is a key player in the formation of mood-controlling neurotransmitters in the brain, it indirectly controls levels of depression. As previously discussed, the cells of depressed individuals are often either unable to properly receive the necessary neurotransmitters, or are unable to correctly perform reuptake of these chemicals, which is also necessary for regulating mood. In addition, depressed people often have too little of the building blocks (amines) needed to create these neurotransmitters.

Through methylation, SAMe converts L-dopa into the neurotransmitter dopamine, and produces the hormone adrenaline. Adequate levels of both these substances are needed to maintain an elevated mood. Moreover, SAMe helps to increase neurotransmitter receptor sensitivity, further warding off depression.

Clinical studies have also shown SAMe to be effective in balancing brain function during drug rehabilitation, and in easing the symptoms of migraine headaches, dementia, and nerve damage.

Treating Depression with SAMe

It is true that SAMe is present in many of the living organisms that we consume. However, it is found in such small amounts, and in such unstable forms, that it cannot be assimilated into the body. Hence, a supplement program using the patented, stabilized form of SAMe now available is your best bet.

It is wise to ease into a dosage program, to decrease the chances of any side effects. Start with a dose of 200 mg per day for two days. On the third day, the dose can be increased to 400 mg taken twice per day. After two weeks have passed, the dose can be raised to 400 mg taken three times per day, and, if needed, 400 mg can be taken four times per day after four weeks. Once symptom relief has been achieved, dosage should be cut back to a reasonable maintenance dose of about 200–400 mg taken once or twice per day.

SAMe should be taken on an empty stomach to enhance absorption. It is most effective in enteric-coated tablet form.

What to Expect when Taking SAMe

The length of time it takes before feeling relief depends on the severity of the condition being treated and the amount of SAMe being taken. Although some individuals feel a difference within one week, it may take a full four-week trial period for SAMe to really kick in.

Clinical studies have shown that SAMe is very safe and rarely causes side effects. The few unwanted effects of oral SAMe supplementation have been nausea, gastrointestinal disturbances, headache, anxiety, and insomnia. These conditions affected a very small percentage of individuals taking higher doses, and they were usually not severe enough to cause a discontinuation of use.

Because SAMe makes liver function more efficient, it appears that it may speed up the clearance of some drugs in the body. However, this has not proven to be a problem. No other drug interactions have been discovered.

CHAPTER 5

KAVA

For centuries, the people of the South Pacific islands have used the healing properties in their native kava plant to bring about feelings of contentment and relaxation. Traditionally, the roots of this bitter-tasting plant were used to make a ceremonial drink that was drunk out of coconut shells in a communal hut. Today, this herb is cultivated on a commercial level and is successfully used in the treatment of anxiety and depression.

What Is Kava?

Kava, or *Piper methysticum,* is a leafy green plant that thrives in the tropical climates of Hawaii, Papua New Guinea, Fiji, and other places in the South Pacific. For 3,000 years, peoples of the South Pacific have relied on kava for cultural and medicinal practices. Traditionally used to settle upset stomachs, soothe insect bites, relieve headaches, fight fungal bacteria, and more, kava is now most well known for its ability to ease anxiety and bring about a feeling of relaxation.

Kava
A plant native to the South Pacific known for its relaxing qualities.

Along with starch, fiber, sugar, proteins, and minerals, there are active ingredients in kava known as kavalactones (or kavapyrones), which are stored in the roots of the plant. Clinical studies have shown that a combination of all of these elements can clear the area around brain receptors for gamma amino butyric acid (GABA). This allows more GABA to bind, resulting in relaxed muscles and relief from anxiety and pain. Furthermore, kavalactones also act on the part of the brain called the amygdala, which controls emotions, heart rate, blood pressure, body temperature, appetite, and more.

Standard antianxiety drugs like benzodiazepines, which include Xanax and Valium, work by mimicking the actions of GABA. Although these chemicals bring about a relaxed feeling, they often cloud thinking, cause sleepiness, slow reaction time, and become addictive. In contrast, kava is nonaddictive and, at regular doses, has no strong side effects.

Using Kava to Treat Depression

Many people who suffer from depression also experience frequent bouts of anxiety. For this reason, kava is useful for replacing anxiety with relaxation, and for helping to restore balance to one's life. In addition, kava is effective in relieving many symptoms of depression such as irritability, pain, and loss of libido.

It is recommended that kava not be used while taking prescription depression or anxiety drugs. If you wish to switch from your current medication to a more natural treatment such as kava, be sure to do it with the help of your physician.

Taking 70–210 mg of kavalactones each day should bring about the desired effects. Experiment to find the minimum dosage for symptom relief. Since many supplements contain only 100 mg of extract, you may need to take several doses during the day to achieve the desired effect. Kava appears to be more potent when taken

Kavalactones
The active ingredients in kava that boost the brain's use of GABA to ease anxiety and pain.

on an empty stomach, although it isn't essential. The total dose of kavalactones should not exceed 300 mg daily.

The active ingredients in kava are most commonly distilled into tinctures, or dried and made into capsules or tablets. High quality products are standardized to a kavalactone content of 30 to 70 percent.

Side Effects Associated with Kava

At high doses, kava can bring about a sleepy or heavily sedated feeling. In addition, extended use of high doses can cause kava dermopathy, a flaky skin condition that usually appears on the palms and the soles of the feet. However, simply reducing dosage can reverse both of these side effects.

Pregnant and nursing women are advised not to take kava. In addition, the effects of this herb on infants and children are not yet known, thus it is recommended that they refrain from its use. Furthermore, kava has been shown to intensify the symptoms of Parkinson's disease, so individuals suffering from this condition should avoid taking this herb.

The Safety of Kava

Over the past five years, a number of cases of liver damage have been reported by kava users. However, no direct correlation has been found between kava use itself and such liver problems. In many of these cases, conventional over-the-counter pharmaceutical drugs with known or potential liver toxicity were also being used.

Until it is certain that kava use is in no way dangerous, the FDA has issued a warning that those individuals with liver problems or who are taking drugs that can harm the liver should check with their physician before taking kava.

Like all treatments for depression or anxiety, kava should be used in combination with other positive steps, such as lifestyle changes. Although long-term, low-dose use of kava has not indicated any negative effects, it would be wise to not use kava continuously for more than four weeks without seeking the advice of a health practitioner.

CHAPTER 6

5-HTP

We now understand that many mood disorders, including depression, are related to a shortage of the brain chemical serotonin. Unfortunately, supplemental serotonin is unable to pass through the blood-brain barrier and therefore cannot be used directly as a supplement. However, supplementing with the precursor to serotonin known as 5-hydroxytryptophan (5-HTP) can bring about improvements in mood. In fact, research has shown that adding 5-HTP to the diet is an effective treatment for depression and anxiety, as well as obesity and premenstrual syndrome.

What Is 5-HTP?

The substance 5-hydroxytryptophan is naturally created in the body from the essential amino acid tryptophan. Tryptophan, present in certain meats, fish, dairy products, and legumes, is transported to the brain via the blood. Once inside the brain, it is acted upon by the enzyme tryptophan hydroxylase and converted into 5-HTP. Then, a second enzyme converts 5-HTP into the neurotransmitter serotonin, a key player in anxiety, attention, aggression, arousal, and thought.

True, boosting the body's level of tryptophan is one way to increase the amount of serotonin in the brain. Unfortunately, supplemental tryptophan is no longer available in the United States except by special prescription. The reason for this is that in 1989 tryptophan was removed from the market because several cases of a muscular condition known as eosinophilia-myalgia were linked to its use. However, it was later discovered that the individuals suffering from this condition had all consumed a specific brand of tryptophan supplement made by the Japanese company Showa Denko. Tests showed that this particular supplement had been manufactured using a process that allowed trace contaminants to enter into the final product. Additional evidence points to the fact that these trace contaminants were responsible for the eosinophilia-myalgia, rather than tryptophan itself.

Certain meats do contain relatively high amounts of tryptophan, however, these foods are also full of other amino acids, so an unwanted balance of amino acids is created in the blood. Eating carbohydrates is actually a better way to increase tryptophan levels in the body, because the insulin released after carbohydrate consumption causes certain amino acids to leave the blood, thus elevating the level of tryptophan.

For most depressed individuals, however, dietary increases in tryptophan will not create high enough levels to increase serotonin in the brain. Fortunately, supplementing the diet directly with 5-HTP—rather than using tryptophan, which is then converted into 5-HTP—makes the process of creating serotonin one step faster.

Using 5-HTP to Treat Depression

In places like Ghana and the Ivory Coast of Africa, there grows a shrubby tree that produces griffonia seeds. These small seeds contain 5 to 10 percent 5-HTP. Once used only by the locals to soothe overexcited children, the seeds are now harvested by vitamin companies for the worldwide production of 5-HTP supplements.

As with most supplements, finding the perfect dose is a process of trial and error. It is best to start with a low dose of 5-HTP, such as 25 mg. If symptoms persist, increase dose by 25-mg increments until reaching 100 mg. Although much higher doses have been safely used to treat severe muscular contractions, the long-term studies of these high doses have not yet been published. Hence, it is recommended to consult a physician before taking doses higher than 100 mg.

Although there are some individuals still not convinced of 5-HTP's safety, the available evidence supports the belief that not only is 5-HTP safe, but it can be used with only infrequent, mild side effects such as sleepiness, nausea, and reduced sex drive. However, as with any supplement, there is always a level of risk. For that reason it is best to read all the available literature and seek the guidance of a physician or nutritionist before beginning a new supplement regimen. A good idea is to try 5-HTP for no more than three months, taking a break for a few days after two to four weeks of supplementation. After that, your health care provider can restart the 5-HTP if needed. To be on the safe side, skip taking 5-HTP one or two days a week.

Individuals who are currently taking serotonin-altering drugs such as antidepressants, L-dopa, or other medications should consult a physician before taking 5-HTP. Moreover, pregnant women and people suffering from other medical conditions should only take 5-HTP under the supervision of a doctor.

Taking 5-HTP with Vitamin B$_6$

Many 5-HTP supplements include vitamin B$_6$ because it is a cofactor in the eventual conversion of tryptophan to serotonin. However, some experts believe taking vitamin B_6 in conjunction with 5-HTP to be counterproductive. Although vitamin B_6 makes 5-HTP conversion in the brain more efficient, it also makes its conversion in the blood more effective—a consequence that ideally should be minimized so that as much 5-HTP as possible reaches the brain intact. The best advice is to try taking 5-HTP with and without vitamin B_6. It is often recommended to take a B-complex supplement in the morning with breakfast, and then take 5-HTP a few hours later.

CHAPTER 7

VITAMINS, MINERALS, AND OTHER NUTRIENTS

Cutting-edge scientific research has now revealed that many people suffering from depression have low levels of certain vitamins such as B_1, B_{12}, C, folic acid, and niacin, as well as deficiencies of minerals such as magnesium and zinc. Since these vitamins and minerals play a major part in the creation and maintenance of mood-regulating neurotransmitters in the brain, as well as in many chemical reactions in the body, their supplementation is a key to treating depression. For many individuals, simply boosting levels of these vitamins is all it takes to improve mood.

Vitamins and a Healthy Diet

Many foods do contain high levels of certain vitamins. For example, organ meats such as kidney and liver are high in the B vitamins, while leafy green vegetables are good sources of folic acid. However, the average American diet—low in complex carbohydrates and high in fat and refined sugar—is deficient in numerous vitamins and minerals, which can affect mood. Even individuals who eat a healthy balanced diet have difficulty meeting the optimum vitamin and mineral levels needed to promote

Recommended Dietary Allowances (RDA)

The minimum daily amounts of vitamins and minerals needed for an adult to prevent diseases that are caused by vitamin deficiencies.

health, which are quite a bit higher than the Recommended Dietary Allowances listed on food products in the United States (which are simply the minimum levels needed to ward off illness). Therefore, in addition to eating a healthy balanced diet, it is highly recommended that one supplement with certain vitamins and minerals.

The Role of the B Vitamins

The B vitamins can have a dramatic influence on mood. These nutrients work together as a team to assist in important functions such as mood regulation, energy metabolism, and the creation of red blood cells. Although each B vitamin has functions specific to itself, they work best when taken together to maximize their synergy and to avoid unwanted effects.

Synergy
The interaction of discrete entities such that their overall effect is greater than the sum of their individual effects would be.

Since the B vitamins work synergistically, it is best to take a basic B complex along with any extra individual B-vitamin supplements. In addition, you should take the active coenzyme form of the B vitamins. Although each supplement regime must be tailored to the individual, some safe, effective dosages are listed below, and are summarized in a chart at the end of this chapter.

The Role of Vitamin B_1

Perhaps the most important role of vitamin B_1 (thiamin) is helping the body burn glucose, amino acids, and fat. Vitamin B_1 also plays an important role in nerve stimulation, in the synthesis of certain brain neurotransmitters, and in the proper function of the adrenal glands, which ultimately control mental and physical stress. Low levels of B_1 have been associated with anxiety, fatigue, depression, poor memory, muscle weakness, vi-

sion problems, and the feeling of pins and nee-
dles in the feet.

Foods such as whole grains, egg yolks, fresh
beans, pork, and brewer's yeast contain relatively
high amounts of vitamin B_1.

As stated earlier, the B vitamins should be
taken together to produce the best results. A
B complex with a daily dose of 100–200 mg of
vitamin B_1 should be sufficient. Potential side
effects from taking vitamin B_1 include gastric
distress and an increase in blood pressure.

The Role of Vitamin B_2

Like the other B vitamins, vitamin B_2 (riboflavin) is
critical to the proper functioning of brain cells.
This nutrient is also important in the metabolism
of essential fatty acids and the quenching of free
radicals in the body. Eating more whole grains,
soybeans, green leafy vegetables, legumes, and
yogurt will provide more B_2. In addition, a supplement that contains 25–50 mg per day is ideal.

The Role of Vitamin B_3

Vitamin B_3, also known as niacin or niacinamide,
produces energy in the body by breaking down
carbohydrates, fats, and proteins. Low levels of
this vitamin have been linked to depression and
anxiety. One reason for this may be that niacin is
a product of tryptophan. Thus, if there are low
levels of tryptophan in the body—as is common
in depressed individuals—then the small supply
available gets used for niacin production rather
than mood-stabilizing serotonin production. Vitamin B_3 supplementation has proven effective in
treating even severe types of depression such as
schizophrenia.

To consume more vitamin B_3 in your diet, eat
organ meats such as kidney and liver, whole
grains, and legumes.

The optimum dose of vitamin B_3 is usually 50–150 mg per day. There are two types of vitamin B_3 on the market, the niacin and the niacinamide forms. Although both forms are effective, high doses of niacinamide can cause itching, nausea, rises in blood sugar, and skin flushing. Although this flush may be startling, it is not dangerous, and can usually be reduced by taking niacin with meals or cold beverages.

Niacin Flush
A harmless reddening of the skin or burning sensation, caused by high doses of niacinamide, which dissipates with regular use.

At doses less than 200 mg per day, the niacin form of B_3 has rarely demonstrated any negative effects. However, potential side effects include headache, vomiting, darkening of the skin, itchiness, and restlessness.

The Role of Vitamin B_6

Vitamin B_6 is one of the most important nutrients for the regulation of mood, because it plays a role in the synthesis of neurotransmitters. In addition, this vitamin is needed for amino acid metabolism, for the absorption of amino acids from the gastrointestinal tract, for carbohydrate and fat metabolism, and for the creation of red blood cells and antibodies.

Deficiencies of vitamin B_6 have been linked to fatigue, anemia, gastrointestinal distress, and neurological symptoms such as seizures, as well as slow wound healing and depression. Studies have shown that alcohol consumption, stress, tobacco use, birth control pills, pregnancy, and antibiotics can contribute to B_6 deficiency.

Besides relieving many of the common symptoms of depression, B_6 supplementation has been found to ease the low moods and other symptoms associated with PMS. In a recent review of nine randomized, double-blind, placebo-controlled B_6 studies published in the *British Medical Journal,* researchers discovered that supplementation with this vitamin significantly improved PMS-related depression, as well as most other PMS symptoms.

Vitamin B_6 can be found in relatively high doses in chicken, beef, fish, eggs, carrots, spinach, avocado, bananas, whole wheat, and alfalfa. But food sources cannot usually provide optimum levels of this nutrient, and supplementation is required.

As mentioned earlier, it is important to take vitamin B_6 in conjunction with the other B vitamins, and to take them in relatively similar proportions. A daily dose of 25–100 mg of vitamin B_6 should be sufficient. Larger doses of B_6 have been useful in treating various kinds of depression, although it is important to work with a trained practitioner when choosing a dose higher than 100 mg.

The Role of Vitamin B_{12}

Vitamin B_{12} is important in the production of energy from fats and sugars, in the health and maintenance of the nervous system, in the production of nucleic acids, which are the building blocks of genes, and in the manufacture of the neurotransmitter acetylcholine.

Low levels of vitamin B_{12} have been associated with symptoms such as difficulty concentrating, mental fatigue, pale complexion, numbness in the toes, anemia, neurological problems, and low moods to severe depression. Your chances of suffering from B_{12} deficiency increase if you are a strict vegetarian, abuse alcohol or other drugs, are under a great deal of stress, have recently undergone surgery, or are suffering from a chronic wasting illness.

Animal products such as milk, cheese, fish, and meat are good sources of vitamin B_{12}. However, the body is only able to absorb about one percent of the total vitamin B_{12} taken in through the diet or supplements. For this reason, B_{12} injections seem to be the most efficient means of absorption; however, they are difficult to acquire.

Therefore, the sublingual form of the vitamin—which is dissolved under the tongue—is usually your best option, because it is taken in through the nearby blood vessels, rather than being slowly absorbed in the stomach.

Many researchers have reaped impressive results using megadoses of B_{12}. In general, however, 500–2,000 mcg of sublingual B_{12} should compensate for any deficiency.

Is Inositol a B Vitamin?

Inositol is a naturally occurring isomer of glucose, which is often classified as part of the vitamin B complex. It is both manufactured in the body and ingested via foods like unprocessed grains, citrus fruits (except lemons), brewer's yeast, wheat germ, lima beans, raisins, peanuts, and lecithin. The nutrient plays a part in maintaining the structure and integrity of cell membranes. In addition, inositol is needed for serotonin to properly bind to its receptors.

Inositol deficiencies have been documented in numerous cases of depression, and have been linked to symptoms of eczema, constipation, eye problems, hair loss, and elevations of cholesterol. A study published in 1978 by Barkai and colleagues showed that both unipolar and bipolar depressed patients had markedly reduced levels of inositol in their cerebrospinal fluid. When eleven of these patients were given 6 g of inositol a day for four weeks, nine of them demonstrated significant improvement. No side effects were observed. Further studies have found similar results. It appears that inositol supplementation is effective in the spectrum of illnesses responsive to SSRIs, including depression, panic, and obsessive-compulsive disorders.

Supplemental inositol should be taken in combination with the other B vitamins. A therapeutic dose of 250–500 mg, two or three times a day, should bring about the desired results.

Inositol use by children, especially those with attention deficit disorder with hyperactivity, should be under the guidance of a physician. Furthermore, individuals suffering from manic-depression should seek the guidance of a medical professional before beginning an inositol supplementation program.

The Role of Folic Acid

Time and time again, studies have shown a strong connection between folic acid deficiency and depression. This vitamin may only be needed in very small amounts, but it is a key player in several important bodily functions. Besides contributing to the formation of norepinephrine and serotonin in the brain, folic acid is important in the synthesis of DNA and RNA, in the production of red blood cells, and in the secretion of hormones. Furthermore, this vitamin works closely with B_6 to sustain low levels of homocysteine, a byproduct of protein metabolism that can lead to cardiovascular disease.

Folic acid deficiency can lead to poor antibody production, anemia, fatigue, memory problems, damaged DNA, and depression. In a 1984 study conducted by Botez and colleagues, folic acid therapy was administered to forty-nine depressed patients: twelve suffering from folate neuropathy and thirty-seven with neurological disorders. The patients showed significant im-

DNA

A complex protein within cells that carries genetic information.

provements in cognitive functioning following one year of folate therapy.

Leafy green vegetables, asparagus, oranges, bananas, pineapples, and organ meats are good sources of dietary folic acid. However, this vitamin is sensitive to heat, so food sources that are cooked may lose some of their vitamin supply. Hence, it is wise to take a folic acid supplement. Considering how little folic acid is needed for optimum health, it is surprising to learn that it is the most common vitamin deficiency in the world. The recommended daily dose is 400–1,000 mcg per day.

The Role of Vitamin C

Vitamin C is most well known for its ability to enhance the immune system. It does this by increasing the activity of virus-killing cells such as white blood cells, T cells, and antibodies. In addition, vitamin C has been proven to be a powerful antioxidant—cleaning up free radicals in the body. Vitamin C also plays an important role in the formation and preservation of norepinephrine and serotonin in the brain, which help to control moods. Furthermore, it is needed for the stimulation of the adrenal glands, a response that is intensified during times of stress.

The proper dosage of vitamin C varies from person to person. Most people achieve the desired results from dosages of 1,000–2,000 mg per day. Test your limit using "bowel tolerance" as a guide—take a divided dose of vitamin C several times a day until your stools become loose. Then, reduce your dose slightly.

It is highly recommended that you take a vitamin C supplement containing bioflavonoids, nutrients that increase the body's ability to absorb vitamin C. Bioflavonoids cannot be produced by the body, but are crucial to the health of brain tissue and the maintenance of brain chemicals. Although it is possible to ingest the recommended dose of bioflavonoids through the diet, supplemental doses of these nutrients have been shown to promote better memory and reduce insomnia. Bioflavonoids are found in citrus, green peppers, broccoli, tomatoes, papayas, cherries, apricots, and grapes.

Minerals Affect Mood, Too

Deficiencies in minerals such as magnesium, calcium, zinc, and iron can have distinct effects on mood. Not only do these minerals play their own important roles in the body, but many of them are necessary in order for vitamins to work effectively. And, like vitamins, many minerals are necessary to catalyze the physiologic reactions in the body.

The Role of Magnesium

Magnesium is a coenzyme needed to form brain neurotransmitters and to metabolize amino acids and carbohydrates. In addition, magnesium is necessary for the proper use of vitamins C and E, and for the conversion of the B vitamins into forms the body can use.

Deficiencies of magnesium can lead to depression, anxiety, restlessness, insomnia, irritability, and hallucinations. Studies have shown your chances of being deficient in magnesium increase if you are under a good deal of stress, suffer from high blood pressure or heart disease, consume lots of alcohol or caffeine, take oral contraceptives, or are pregnant.

Many foods serve as good sources of this mineral, such as raw almonds, sesame seeds, brewer's yeast, wheat germ, oats, rye, peas, carrots, and beet greens. Most individuals benefit from 400–800 mg of magnesium per day. This mineral should be taken in conjunction with vitamin B_6 for proper absorption. The most readily absorbed forms of this mineral are the orotate and aspartate forms.

Individuals suffering from kidney failure, Addison's disease, or myasthemia granis should check with their physician before taking magnesium supplements.

The Role of Zinc

Although the body requires only small amounts of this mineral, it is critical to proper brain function. Zinc deficiencies have been linked to physical as well as psychological disorders.

Seek out zinc-rich foods such as organ and red meats, whole grains, and shellfish, especially if you suffer from an eating disorder, high estrogen levels, diabetes, or anemia. In addition, because zinc and copper naturally strive to balance each other in the body, an excess of copper in the diet can create a zinc deficit.

Most often, 15–50 mg of zinc per day is sufficient to maintain optimum health. Doses of 100 mg or more of this mineral taken for extended periods of time have been shown to cause depletions in copper and iron.

The Role of Iron

Most people are aware of the toll iron deficiency can reap on the body. The weakness, lethargy, and depression caused by low levels of iron are due in part to a lack of oxygen in the blood. That is because iron is part of hemoglobin, the oxygen-carrying component of the blood. Adequate levels of iron are also necessary for the proper metabolism of the B vitamins, as well as for the formation of brain neurotransmitters. Thus, iron affects mood regulation in two ways.

Depression can result from an excess of iron as

well. A study published in the *Canadian Journal of Psychiatry* found that treating seven depressed patients with chelation therapy reduced their iron overload and, subsequently, improved their depression. Since oversupplementation of iron can lead to toxicity, it is recommended that men and postmenopausal women do not supplement their diet with iron on its own. Instead, find a multivitamin that includes 5–15 mg of iron.

When to Use Supplements

Remember, you don't have to be suffering from severe deficiencies to benefit from nutrient supplementation. Although nutrient level testing is not common medical practice, you can request that your health practitioner test you for deficiencies. Testing is especially important if you suffer from a number of the following symptoms: depression, skin disorders, lesions around or in the mouth, numbness in the extremities, dizziness, or hair loss.

Recommended Daily Supplement Doses for Treating Depression

- Vitamin B_1:   100–200 mg
- Vitamin B_2:   25–50 mg
- Vitamin B_3:   50–150 mg
- Vitamin B_6:   25–100 mg
- Vitamin B_{12}:   500–2,000 mcg
- Vitamin C: 1,000–2,000 mg
- Inositol: 250–500 mg
- Folic acid: 400–1,000 mg
- Magnesium: 400–800 mg
- Zinc: 15–50 mg
- Iron: 5–15 mg

CHAPTER 8

MELATONIN

Supplementation with the hormone melatonin has been shown to improve sleep, combat free radicals, and relieve depression and other mood disorders. That is because this hormone helps regulate the body's internal clock and, in so doing, succeeds in creating a chemical balance in the brain and thus a feeling of improved well-being.

What Is Melatonin?

Melatonin, or N-acetyl-5-methoxyserotonin, is a naturally occurring hormone produced in a small organ at the base of the brain called the pineal gland, as well as in the large intestine and the retina of the eye. Although humans produce melatonin throughout their lifetime, levels of this hormone reach their peak during adolescence and decrease thereafter.

The production of this hormone occurs mainly at night and in light-free environments. In fact, the making of melatonin is what signals to the body that it is time to sleep. In the morning, when daylight reaches our eyes, melatonin production ceases, and the body begins to make hormones that control other bodily activities.

How Melatonin Functions in the Body

The most well known of melatonin's functions is the maintenance of the body's biological clock, which is responsible for tasks such as elevating

Biological Clock
Self-regulating functions of the body that follow cyclical patterns and control sleep and wakefulness, body temperature, blood pressure, the production of hormones, and other processes.

mood, regulating sleep, and controlling appetite. Melatonin also has been shown to work as a powerful antioxidant, to stimulate the immune system, to work as a painkiller, and to alleviate jet lag.

In addition, melatonin is closely linked to the mood-regulating neurotransmitter serotonin. This neurotransmitter is responsible for neuropsychological functions such as memory, appetite, and mood. When levels of one of these two substances drops, so do levels of the other. Thus, melatonin is a key player in mood regulation.

Melatonin Supplements Elevate Mood

Studies dating as far back as the early 1970s reveal that individuals who were given melatonin to alleviate jet lag or to induce sleep discovered additional feelings of contentment and improved mood. More recently, research into the mechanism behind melatonin's effects has shown that it functions in the same way as standard MAO inhibitors such as Nardil or Parnate. These drugs prevent the substance monoamine oxidase from breaking down serotonin, dopamine, and norepinephrine, thus increasing their supply and improving mood. Furthermore, these antidepressants naturally increase melatonin levels in the body, suggesting that melatonin plays a key role in mood regulation.

Since melatonin levels are closely tied to serotonin levels, it appears that mild to moderate depression may be an indicator of melatonin deficiency. Moreover, melatonin deficiencies have been associated with disruptions in sleep patterns, the occurrence of gray hairs, weight gain, and increased frequency of colds.

As mentioned above, the level of melatonin in the body decreases over time. Although most healthy individuals under the age of forty produce adequate levels of melatonin, there are some conditions that have been linked to melatonin deficiency. For example, stressful lifestyles can lead to an abundance of free radicals in the body, which can reduce melatonin production. In addition, alcohol, caffeine, sleep deprivation, and radiation exposure have also been shown to deplete levels of melatonin. If you suspect you may be melatonin-deficient, ask your doctor to check your blood levels of this hormone.

How Much Melatonin Do I Need?

Finding the correct dose of a supplement is often an exercise in trial and error, and it is always wise to seek the guidance of a health professional when beginning a new supplement program. In the case of melatonin, factors such as your age, your individual body chemistry, the reason for taking melatonin, the type of supplement you choose, and the health of your liver ultimately determine how much you need. For these reasons it is best to begin with a very low dose, such as 0.1 mg, and build up if necessary. Generally, a 3-mg dose will induce sleep-related hormonal activities within two hours of ingestion. This should feel as though your natural body clock is at work. Then, during the night, the increase in melatonin will allow you to sleep more deeply than without supplements. If your goal is to alleviate jet lag, doses of 1–10 mg just before bedtime (local time) should do the trick.

It is common for people taking melatonin to experience more vivid dreams. This appears to be because melatonin extends the nightly periods of REM sleep—the section of the sleep cycle when dreams occur.

Is Melatonin Safe?

Clinical studies have shown no serious side effects in conjunction with melatonin supplementation. Occasionally, large doses of this hormone have brought about mild effects such as daytime sleepiness or sleeplessness during the night.

While melatonin appears to be safe, it is important to remember that it is a powerful hormone that can affect many bodily processes. It is recommended that individuals who are trying to become pregnant, are pregnant or breastfeeding, are taking prescription medication, are contending with kidney disease, or who have an autoimmune disease should consult a physician before taking melatonin.

CHAPTER 9

LIGHT THERAPY

Although people who are depressed be-cause of melatonin deficiencies find that their moods are improved by melatonin supple-ments, a different group of people suffer from ex-cessive amounts of melatonin in the body. This condition, known as seasonal affective disorder (SAD), is a specific type of depression caused by a lack of sunlight exposure. When the body is deprived of sunlight due to seasonal weather changes, swing-shift work hours, or too much time indoors, an excess of melatonin is pro-duced, and frequently, an imbalance of the neu-rotransmitters serotonin and dopamine occurs as well. Melatonin produces feelings of slug-gishness and sleepiness. Treatment with high-intensity lights has proven to be effective in the treatment of SAD.

What Is Seasonal Affective Disorder?

This form of depression is the re-sult of high melatonin and low serotonin levels due to a defi-ciency of sunlight. In areas of the world where winter months bring short, dark days, there is a high prevalence of this condition. The symptoms of SAD include anxiety, sadness, fa-tigue, headaches, short attention span, overeat-ing, and a craving for carbohydrates.

SAD
Seasonal affective disorder, a deficiency of serotonin caused by lack of sunlight.

In addition to nutritional and herbal therapies,

many SAD sufferers can be treated using light therapy. This technique involves exposure to intense levels of light in a controlled environment. The patient sits in front of a box consisting of a set of 2,500–10,000 lux fluorescent bulbs with a diffusing screen. With his or her head and body oriented toward the light, the patient can read, eat, or write while absorbing the powerful rays. Treatment sessions last from fifteen minutes to three hours, once or twice a day, depending on the individual's needs and equipment used.

The Science behind Light Therapy

The body's internal clock, which controls daily rhythms such as temperature, hormone secretion, and sleep patterns, is light-sensitive. When little light is taken in through the eyes, production of melatonin increases, signaling the body to sleep. Internal processes slow down. When ambient light increases, production of melatonin slows down or ceases, and the body becomes alert.

Researchers around the country and abroad have had great success in treating SAD patients with light therapy. For example, scientists at Columbia-Presbyterian Medical Center in New York City found that, of one hundred SAD patients who used a 10,000-lux system for thirty minutes a day, three-quarters of them showed major improvement in depressive symptoms. Further experiments showed that some patients require even less exposure to reap the same benefits.

Although brightening your work or living environment with additional lighting may help you feel more awake, studies show that most SAD sufferers require exposure to the sunlike light levels that only high-intensity lamps provide. Suppliers of these lamps can be found in the resource section.

Side Effects of Light Treatment

There have been very few side effects linked to light therapy. A small percentage of patients experience headaches, eye irritation, or nausea. However, these symptoms are mild and tend to dissipate after a few days. There have been a few cases of patients feeling overly stimulated after receiving treatments. Symptoms such as insomnia, restlessness, and irritability should be discussed with a skilled light-therapy clinician.

Light therapy systems are designed to screen out the ultraviolet light that causes tanning. Occasionally, however, individuals with extremely sensitive skin will show reddening under these lights, in which case extra filters or sunscreen can be used.

Clinical studies have not involved individuals suffering from ocular or retinal pathologies such as glaucoma, retinopathy, cataracts, or retinal detachment. Although no adverse effects have been seen in the eye health of light therapy patients, caution is warranted for those with extremely sensitive skin. In addition, there have yet to be long-term studies of the effects of light therapy on pregnant women, although no hazard is suspected.

CHAPTER 10

FOOD AND DEPRESSION

We all know that the old saw is true: we are what we eat. However, many people do not realize that what they choose to eat can have an almost immediate effect on their daily physiology and mood. This is because certain foods greatly influence the levels of brain chemicals needed for mood regulation. By excluding or minimizing the intake of substances like sugar, caffeine, and alcohol, you can drastically increase your feelings of health and well-being. Likewise, adding high-energy foods to your diet such as certain animal products, soy foods, nuts, and legumes can stimulate the brain and produce energy in the body.

How Foods Affect Brain Chemicals

Specific amino acids such as tyrosine or tryptophan—which are contained in certain meats, fish, dairy products, and legumes—are converted into proteins by the body. These proteins are then further synthesized into brain chemicals like serotonin, which, as we have seen, plays a key role in anxiety, attention, aggression, arousal, mood, and thought.

Surprisingly, the rate at which tryptophan is converted into serotonin depends on the amount of carbohydrates consumed. Blood levels of tryptophan are increased with the ingestion of carbohydrate foods. This increase in blood tryptophan leads to an increase in serotonin production, and for many people, this brings about a feeling of well-being or calm. For other people, however, carbohydrate foods can cause sleepiness.

How Sugar Changes Mood

Studies have shown that people who crave carbohydrates and sugar have a high susceptibility to clinical depression. Since many of these individuals are suffering from low levels of serotonin, eating carbohydrates can often relieve feelings of tension and anxiety temporarily. Thus, for some people, carbohydrate food cravings are a way to elevate neurotransmitters and control mood.

Sugar, a simple carbohydrate, can have many druglike effects on the body, and is considered addictive by many health care professionals. When refined carbohydrates or sugars are ingested, blood sugar levels increase almost immediately. This signals the pancreas to release the hormone insulin, which causes blood sugar levels to drop back down—usually below normal levels. At this point, growth hormone—made of glucagon, cortisol, and adrenaline—pours into the system to help re-elevate blood sugar. In response to this increase, insulin is released once again and the cycle continues. This is the physiological explanation for sugar highs and lows.

Sugar High
A sharp rise in blood sugar due to the ingestion of refined carbohydrates or sugar.

Moderate to high consumption of sugar has been shown to prevent the absorption of certain nutrients, including the B vitamins and some amino acids. Furthermore, sugar has been proven to aggravate certain types of arthritis and asthma, promote tooth decay and yeast infections, raise blood lipid levels, weaken the immune system, and create mood fluctuations.

Hypoglycemia

Hypoglycemia is a condition that may be brought on by the consumption of too much sugar or refined carbohydrates. Individuals suffering from hypoglycemia do not metabolize blood sugar normally, which leaves them with a lower than normal blood sugar level. To compensate for this, many of these individuals give in to carbohydrate cravings, which triggers the blood sugar–insulin roller coaster described above. Up to 77 percent of people who have low blood sugar also suffer from depression. Furthermore, brain scans of depressed patients have proven that low blood sugar or rapidly changing sugar levels affect brain function, and thus moods and emotional states.

Hypoglycemia
The inability to metabolize blood sugar normally.

When blood sugar drops and hormones go into effect, an individual may suffer from sweating, nervousness, hunger, weakness, and shakes. Individuals who experience frequent low blood sugar often suffer from an array of symptoms such as low energy levels, headaches, insomnia, leg cramps, cravings, nightmares, anxiety, mental confusion, irritability, heart palpitations, depression, and more.

Examining your own eating habits and how you feel in response to them is the best way to determine how your body reacts to sugar. Anyone who regularly eats sugar, drinks alcohol, and suffers from several of the symptoms listed above should see a health practitioner to undergo hypoglycemic testing.

Food Allergies and Depression

Both food allergies and food sensitivities can have a profound impact on the body. At the extreme end of the spectrum, an allergy can cause swelling of the bronchial airways, shock, or even death. But allergies do not have to be violent to cause harm. Bloating, headache, digestive problems, dark circles under the eyes, hives, eczema, acne, joint pain, insomnia, irritability, fatigue, foggy thinking, and depression are all common signs of a food allergy. If you frequently suffer from a number of these symptoms, seek the advice of a health care practitioner or allergist who will help you determine your sensitivities.

The classical definition of a food allergy is an immediate or chronic immune reaction to the ingestion of food, whereas a food sensitivity is a nonimmune response such as an upset stomach, headache, or nausea. Both conditions have also been shown to produce chronic low moods. For example, in a study published in the *Annals of Allergy*, researchers found that depressed individuals had four-and-a-half times as many antibody reactions to a set number of foods and inhalants as did nondepressed individuals. Additional studies have revealed that individuals with specific food sensitivities, such as lactose intolerance or an inability to digest the sugar in fruit, are significantly more depressed than those without such sensitivities.

> **Food Sensitivity**
> An allergic reaction characterized by low-grade negative physiological responses to the ingestion of a specific food.

Causes of Food Allergies

A number of foods, such as tomatoes and spinach, contain histamines—biological compounds designed to protect the body from foreign molecules, but that cause inflammation, itchiness, mucus, and rashes when released in large numbers. Other foods, including shellfish, milk, eggs and chocolate, cause the body to release histamines it has stored in white blood cells. In some individuals, for unknown reasons, the body does not know when to stop this histamine-release, and allergylike symptoms result.

The most common food allergies and sensitivities are to foods that are highly present in the American diet. Wheat, dairy products, corn, soy, and sugar pose the biggest threat, and ironically, they are the foods present in nearly every processed food on the shelf.

Histamine
A compound in the body that in large quantities dilates blood vessels, constricts bronchial tubes, and causes itching and hives.

One sure way to rule out food allergies as a source of depression is to have an allergist test for such reactions. Testing techniques can range from skin and oral transmissions of a potential allergen to antibody-sensitive blood work.

An elimination diet is an at-home testing option. By avoiding all common food allergens for a period of time through a strict cleansing diet or a fast, and then adding suspect foods back to your diet one at a time, it is possible to isolate which food is causing the symptoms and sensitivities. Ask your health practitioner for guidance when starting a fast or elimination diet.

Fats and Depression

In general, the American diet is too high in omega-6 fatty acids, like those contained in safflower, soybean, and corn oils, and too low in the omega-3 fats found in foods like salmon and flaxseed. Such an imbalance has been linked to chronic conditions including diabetes, rheumatoid arthritis, ulcerative colitis, cardiovascular disease—and depression.

Most likely, inadequate levels of dietary fats contribute to depression by impairing the functions of cells, including those in the brain. Without proper fatty acids, these brain cells cannot properly synthesize neurotransmitters, send signal transmissions, uptake serotonin, or allow for neurotransmitter binding—all functions essential to maintaining mood.

Why Essential Fatty Acids are Healthy

The EFAs, consisting of alpha-linolenic acid (omega-3) and linoleic acid (omega-6), are substances necessary to good health that cannot be manufactured by the body and, thus, must be taken in through the diet. It is the highly reactive nature of these fats that makes them so fundamental to bodily functions, and which allows them to increase oxidation and metabolic rate. Furthermore, because their chemical structure contains double bonds, EFAs carry a slight negative charge, which causes them to repel each other. This is why EFAs don't clog arteries and contribute to heart disease the way saturated fats do.

Essential Fatty Acids *Fats that are essential to good health but cannot be manufactured by the body and, thus, must be taken in through the diet.*

The tasks EFAs accomplish in the body are even more important than the ones they don't. For example, these substances are key players in the conversion of food to energy, the transfer of oxygen to cells, the production of hormonelike prostaglandins—which guard against conditions like cancer and heart disease—and the formation and maintenance of cell membranes, including those in the brain.

Fats and the American Diet

The reason why you need omega-3 and omega-6 in ample amounts is because they are used by every cell in the body, and they influence the metabolism of all the cells. If these fatty acids are not in close to equal amounts, and you end up with an excess of omega-6—a common condition due to Americans' overconsumption of safflower, corn, and soybean oils—then you end up with an excess of metabolites in the body. These substances tend to compromise health in a number of ways, such as causing inflammatory reactions and encouraging chronic conditions such as heart disease, hypertension, and depression.

To make matters worse, Americans often further intensify this EFA imbalance by loading up on foods that contain trans-fatty acids. These artery-clogging saturated fats are usually found in processed foods and those that contain hydrogenated oils or margarine, such as fried and baked goods. Trans-fatty acids interfere with the normal function of omega-3 and omega-6 fatty acids.

Trans-Fatty Acids
Artery-clogging fats found in margarine and fried and processed foods.

Balancing EFAs in the Diet

For proper diet, it is very important to avoid trans fats, cut down on safflower, soybean, and corn oils, and begin using oils that are rich in omega-3 fatty acids such as canola, flaxseed, and walnut. Since flaxseed oil has the highest percentage of omega-3, daily supplementation with this oil can help neutralize the effects of both trans-fatty acids and excessively high levels of omega-6.

Remember, however, that once a balance of EFAs has been established in the body, flaxseed oil is not the best choice to maintain it. Long-term exclusive use of flaxseed oil can result in omega-6 deficiency symptoms, because flax contains three times more omega-3 than omega-6. Although it would take years for this deficiency to develop, it is best to vary the oils you use. Try using flaxseed oil for several months to make up for an omega-3 deficiency, then switch to a more balanced oil for maintenance such as hempseed or one of the prepared blends.

Once established, maintaining the proper balance of EFAs is not difficult. In fact, many experts believe the optimum daily dose is only 9–18 grams of omega-6 and 2–9 grams of omega-3, which can take the form of a single tablespoon of flaxseed or hempseed oil in oatmeal in the morning, or a splash of walnut-oil vinaigrette on a lunchtime salad.

Caffeine's Effect on Mood

Caffeine is the most popular drug in the world. Its use affects the brain, nervous system, circulation, heart, digestion, muscular system, and more. In small doses of 65–130 mg, caffeine actually improves physical and mental performance. However, consumption beyond these levels can bring about insomnia, anxiety, trembling muscles, headaches, irregular heartbeat, fatigue, dizziness, weakness, and depression.

Caffeine stimulates the release of certain brain amines such as norepinephrine, which causes the lift in mood we are all so familiar with. However, overconsumption of caffeine can cause a depletion of these amines, leaving us fatigued and nervous. In addition, caffeine interferes with the absorption of B vitamins and zinc, and causes a loss of calcium, sodium, and magnesium. As we have already learned, a deficiency of any one of these nutrients can contribute to mood disorders and depression.

The amount of caffeine that is healthy for an individual to consume is ultimately dependent on body weight and physiology, but sticking to a consumption under 200 mg per day is a good general guideline. Keep in mind that an eight-ounce cup of coffee has 120–240 mg of caffeine, a five-ounce cup of tea has 25–110 mg, and a can of caffeinated soda has 30–50 mg.

Alcohol Consumption and Mood Disorders

First of all, alcohol is a depressant. Second, like sugar and refined carbohydrates, it is nutritionally useless. It is simply empty calories that cannot be converted into energy unless certain vitamins are present in adequate quantities. Furthermore, alcohol consumption has been shown to prevent the proper absorption of the B vitamins and certain amino acids, to destroy vitamins C and B already in the body, and to cause urinary loss of zinc, magnesium, calcium, and vitamin B_{12}. These alcohol-induced deficiencies can certainly lead to mood disorders and depression.

Because it is so addictive, alcohol use can also prevent an individual from confronting the issues contributing to his or her depression. Thus, it can prolong and intensify the depressed state.

In general, alcohol consumption is not beneficial for the body or mind. In fact, recent studies have shown that even small amounts of alcohol can inhibit the proper synthesis of neurotransmitters in the brain. If you do consume alcohol, be sure to enhance your diet with the necessary nutritional supplements. If you are a heavy drinker, cut back or cease your drinking. Get help if you need to.

CHAPTER 11

LIFESTYLE CHOICES

The easiest solution to many people's depression is the one most often overlooked. Besides treating one's depression with supplemental herbs, vitamins, and other nutrients, simple changes in lifestyle can markedly improve health and mood without the need for adding any substances to the body. These quality-of-life choices include getting adequate sleep and exercise, taking the time to relax the body and mind through meditation, and seeking the counseling of a trained therapist or other health practitioner. Making changes in even one of these areas can make a world of difference in the way you feel.

How Much Sleep Does One Really Need?

Although many people claim to need very little sleep, studies have shown that most adults require a good seven hours to function properly. When we don't get adequate sleep, due to stress, anxiety, insomnia, or external factors, it can contribute to a weakened immune system, slowed reflexes, and depression.

Studies have shown that depriving a person of REM sleep for extended periods of time results in various psychotic conditions, including depression. This is due to the fact that sleep deprivation can cause up to a 20

REM Sleep
The Rapid Eye Movement cycle of sleep, when dreaming occurs and many brain functions are regulated.

percent decrease in brain serotonin levels. Ironically, serotonin is needed to initiate REM sleep,
and must be present at certain levels to maintain
this sleep cycle. Thus, low serotonin levels can
cause insomnia, and insomnia in turn can decrease serotonin levels in an ongoing vicious
cycle.

Getting Adequate Rest

Many traditional antidepressant drugs actually inhibit REM sleep and, thus, contribute to sleep
deprivation. For this reason, as well as the many
others that have been discussed throughout this
book, it is often best to deal with one's depression symptoms—such as insomnia—using natural means.

To encourage better sleep, try practicing the
following steps:

1. Get into bed at a reasonable hour.

2. Eliminate sugar, caffeine, and alcohol from
your diet.

3. Practice relaxation techniques such as yoga
and deep breathing.

4. Get adequate exercise during the day.

5. If necessary, supplement your nightly sleep
with a short afternoon nap.

Exercise may be the best way to improve your
sleep. A recent controlled clinical trial involving
thirty-two older adults (ages 60–84) who had
major depression demonstrated that a ten-week
program of weight-training exercise, three times
per week, significantly improved sleep quality
and mood.

A number of herbs have also proven to help
induce sleep by reducing anxiety, including St.
John's wort and kava. A dose of 300 mg of St.

John's wort, taken three times per day, or a daily dose of 120 mg of kava should bring some relief and encourage better sleep.

Exercise and Depression

Not only does regular exercise increase self-esteem, improve sleep, ward off depression, increase energy, and improve concentration, but it also raises serotonin production and activity. In other words, regular exercise can help balance the levels of neurotransmitters that ensure deep sleep and elevated mood. On top of all this, of course, exercise is the best way to improve overall health in the body as well.

The benefits of exercise appear to exist regardless of the specific activity. In one trial, forty depressed women were randomly assigned to eight weeks of running, a weight-lifting program, or no exercise. At the end of the study, members of both exercise groups were less depressed than the control group. The authors concluded that a positive outcome did not depend on the type of activity or the level of physical fitness achieved.

According to governmental recommendations, thirty minutes of exercise a day will help prevent many disease conditions including heart disease, obesity, and depression. This daily exercise can be in the form of everyday activities such as walking, gardening, or vacuuming. While aerobic exercise has been found to be the most effective in increasing energy and maintaining health, it is interesting to note that weight-training was found to be the most beneficial in terms of self-esteem.

The key to effective exercise is finding an activity that you enjoy. Whether it is walking, gardening, or yoga, choosing an activity that you look forward to doing for at least thirty minutes every other day is the best way to keep yourself doing it. It is also important to reach the point of fatigue when exercising in order for serotonin to be produced. It is best not to exercise 2–3 hours before bed, as evening exercise may contribute to sleeplessness.

Exercise is beneficial to the body in so many ways, both mentally and physically, that it is a crime for anyone to avoid it entirely. Get out there and exercise; you'll be surprised how much better you feel.

Staying Social

By nature, humans are social creatures. However, when feelings of depression take hold, many people's desire for social interaction diminishes. This often exacerbates the problem, for a lack of social interaction has been shown to actually promote depression. For these people, cultivating a sense of belonging may be just the thing to lift mood. In fact, researchers at the University of Michigan School of Nursing found that developing close relationships or fitting in to a group greatly reduced the symptoms of depression.

Find a social outlet that feels right for you. Whether it is a cooking class, ski club, spiritual center, or support group, becoming part of a community can certainly help create a sense of belonging and ease feelings of depression.

CHAPTER 12

SEEKING PROFESSIONAL HELP

Perhaps the most important step in treating depression is simply choosing to get help. By reading this book you have made a huge first step in that process. It is highly recommended that you seek the guidance of a trained health practitioner to determine the nature of your depression and the best means of treating it. By working with a practitioner knowledgeable in both standard and natural approaches for treating depression, you will be giving yourself every available option.

Generally, if you are having frequent suicidal thoughts, have been depressed for a considerable period of time, are having trouble sleeping, have lost your appetite, have low energy, or your sadness is interfering with your job, relationships, or health, then it is time to seek professional help. Talking with a friend or family member about these feelings can be a good way to determine the severity of your depression. If you do not have someone to talk with to create such a "reality check," then contacting a health professional is a good choice.

There are organizations listed at the end of this book that can help you locate a health care practitioner who is educated in natural treatments. Be sure to be open about your concerns and desires regarding approaches for treatment. Be patient, and remember that therapy can be an integral part of overcoming depression.

Talk Therapy for Depression

Psychological approaches to treating depression can be highly effective on their own or in conjunction with a number of strategies outlined in this book. Supportive counseling can help ease the pain of depression as well as address its underlying causes.

In general, psychotherapy describes any form of communication between a pyschotherapist and a patient for the purpose of remedying whatever psychological issues the patient needs to resolve. In two studies recently reported in *The Archives of General Psychiatry,* the effects of interpersonal psychotherapy—short-term talk treatment focusing on social relationships—were compared to those of antidepressant drugs. In one of the studies, patients were given either twelve weeks of psychotherapy or twelve weeks of the antidepressant Paxil. Using PET brain scans as a measure of brain function, researchers found that patients who responded to either treatment had nearly identical changes in brain function. In other words, pharmacotherapy and psychotherapy can produce similar effects on brain activity.

Talk therapy may not be the solution for all conditions. It seems ineffective for diseases like schizophrenia. However, it is clear that therapy can improve depression in many cases.

Choosing a Therapist

There are many different styles of psychotherapy, therefore it is important to explore all of your options. While psychiatrists, psychotherapists, and social workers can all serve as therapists, only a psychiatrist can prescribe medication. However, if you are interested in treating your depression naturally, there is no need for a prescription.

The organizations listed at the end of this book are a good place to start when considering therapy. In addition, one's friends, family, and general practitioner can often recommend the names of prospective therapists. Options range from classical psychoanalysis to dance and art therapy, so if your first experience is not the solution, keep trying.

When meeting a therapist for the first time, be sure that he or she is completely focused on you and clearly interested in your problem. An initial visit will most likely include a diagnostic evaluation, which includes questions related to how long you have felt depressed, as well as ones regarding your sleep, eating, and work habits.

By the end of your first visit, you should ask your therapist for a summary of his or her evaluation and what type of therapy he or she recommends. The key to building a working relationship with your therapist is to feel comfortable and safe from the very beginning.

CONCLUSION

It seems criminal that nearly one in three people in this country suffers from some form of depression, especially when you consider that it is one of the most readily treatable conditions. As you have discovered in this book, an array of natural therapies are as effective in relieving depression—and far safer for the body and mind—as are the host of standard antidepressant treatments commonly prescribed.

As the scientific information in this book demonstrates, depression is often linked to brain chemical imbalances, which can usually be corrected through diet modifications, health-promoting herbs and supplements, and simple lifestyle changes. Although it may seem hard to believe that the intense feelings of sadness, fatigue, and hopelessness brought on by depression can be remedied by such simple treatments, the truth is that thousands of people have already succeeded in overcoming depression using these techniques.

You can use the information in this book to jump-start your healing process. Then, continue to educate yourself in these natural treatments, and seek the guidance of a health professional who understands the power of these approaches. By taking these proactive steps, you will soon find the emotional balance, well-being, and love of life you have been missing.

SUPPLEMENT REFERENCE GUIDE

Due to the fact that individual nutrient needs and restrictions vary, it is best to seek the guidance of a trained physician when beginning a supplement treatment program. It is especially important to check with your doctor if you are pregnant, nursing, or taking any medication. The dosages listed below are general guidelines for daily intake. Your needs may differ.

Vitamin B_1

Natural sources: avocado, banana, beans, brewer's yeast, leafy green vegetables

Dosage: 100–200 mg

Safety: Do not take this vitamin with anticonvulsant medications. Consult a physician if you are anemic.

Vitamin B_2

Natural sources: soybeans, leafy green vegetables, nuts, seeds

Dosage: 25–50 mg

Safety: No known safety concerns.

Vitamin B_3

Natural sources: beef liver, peanut butter, salmon, soybeans, tuna

Dosage: 50–150 mg

Safety: Do not take this vitamin if you are suffering from peptic ulcer or impaired

liver function. Consult a physician if you
have diabetes, glaucoma, or gout.

Vitamin B$_6$

Natural sources: lentils, shrimp, sunflower
seeds, wheat germ, chicken

Dosage: 25–100 mg

Safety: Consult a physician if you are suffering
from overactive thyroid, sickle-cell anemia,
or a liver condition.

Vitamin B$_{12}$

Natural sources: beef, dairy products, oysters,
sardines, clams, flounder

Dosage: 500–2,000 mcg

Safety: Consult a physician if you are taking
anticonvulsant medication.

Vitamin C

Natural sources: broccoli, grapefruit, kiwi, kale,
tomatoes

Dosage: 1,000–2,000 mg

Safety: Consult a physician if you are suffering
from gout, kidney stones, or sickle-cell
anemia.

Inositol

Natural sources: cantaloupe, garbanzo beans,
nuts, lentils

Dosage: 250–500 mg

Safety: Consult a physician if you are suffering
from diabetes.

Folic Acid

Natural sources: avocado, bananas, beans,
brewer's yeast, leafy green vegetables, lentils

Dosage: 400–1,000 mg

Safety: Do not take folic acid with anticonvulsant medications. Consult a
   physician if you are anemic.

Magnesium

Natural sources: avocado, leafy green
   vegetables, nuts, shrimp, wheat germ

Dosage: 400–800 mg

Safety: Consult a physician if you are suffering
   from a kidney condition.

Zinc

Natural sources: egg yolk, oysters, molasses,
   sesame seeds, soybeans

Dosage: 15–50 mg

Safety: Consult a physician if you are suffering
   from stomach ulcers.

Iron

Natural sources: egg yolk, lentils, molasses,
   oysters, seaweed

Dosage: 5–15 mg

Safety: Do not take iron if you have acute
   hepatitis. Consult a physician if you have
   a kidney condition.

St. John's wort

Dosage: Begin with 300 mg of an extract
   standardized to 3 percent hyperforin.
   Build up to 900 mg in divided doses.

Safety: Consult a physician if you are pregnant,
   nursing, taking medication, on birth control
   pills, or are scheduled for surgery.

Kava

Dosage: 70–210 mg kavalactones

Safety: Do not use kava if you are taking
   prescription antidepressant or antianxiety

medication. Do not take kava if you have Parkinson's disease or liver problems. Do not exceed 300 mg kavalactones per day.

5-HTP

Dosage: Start with 25 mg and work up to 100 mg.

Safety: Limit use to no more than three consecutive months. Take a break every 2–4 weeks. Skip 1–2 days per week. Do not take 5-HTP if you are on antidepressant drugs, pregnant, or nursing.

SAMe

Dosage: Begin with 200 mg for two days. On the third day take 400 mg two times per day. After two weeks, take 400 mg three times per day. When symptom relief occurs, cut back to 200–400 mg. Take doses on an empty stomach.

Safety: Consult a physician if you are on any medication, pregnant, nursing, or are scheduled for surgery.

Melatonin

Dosage: 0.2–10 mg taken at bedtime to improve sleep. To alleviate jet lag, take 1–10 mg before bed (local time).

Safety: May cause daytime sleepiness. Consult a physician if you are pregnant, nursing, taking medication, or suffering from kidney disease.

SELECTED
REFERENCES

Abou-Saleh, MT, Coppen, A. The biology of folate in depression: implications for nutritional hypotheses of the psychoses. *J Psychiat Res*, 1986; 20(2):91–101.

Adams, PB, Lawson, S, Sanigorski, A, et al. Arachidonic acid to eicosapentaenoic acid ratio in blood correlates positively with clinical symptoms of depression. *Lipids*, 1996; 31(Suppl):S 157–61.

Barnes, J, Anderson, LA, Phillipson, JD. St. John's wort (Hypericum perforatum L.): a review of its chemistry, pharmacology and clinical properties. *J Pharm Pharmacol*, 2001; 53:583–600.

Benjamin, J, Agam, G, Levine J, et al. Inositol treatment in psychiatry. *Psychopharmacology Bulletin*, 1995; 31:167–75.

Dolberg, OT, Hirschmann, S, Grunhaus, L. Melatonin for the treatment of sleep disturbances in major depressive disorder. *Am J Psychiatry*, 1998; 155(8):1119–21.

Ernst, E, Rand, JI, Stevinson, C. Complementary therapies for depression: an overview. *Archives of General Psychiatry*, 1998; 55(11):1026–32.

Head, A, Kendall, MJ, Ferner, R, et al. Acute effects of beta blockade and exercise on mood and anxiety. *Br J Sports Med*, 1996; 30(3):238–42.

Kendell, RE, Wainwright, S, Hailey, A, et al. The influence of childbirth on psychiatric morbidity. *Psychol Med*, 1976; 6(2):297–302.

Kendler, KS, Walters, EE, Truett, KR, et al. Sources of individual differences in depressive symptoms: analysis of two samples of twins and their families. *Am J Psychiatry*, 1994; 51:1605–14.

Linde, K, Ramirez, G, Mulrow, CD, et al. St. John's wort for depression—an overview and meta-analysis of randomized clinical trials. *Br Med J*, 1996; 313:253–58.

Marshall, PS. Allergy and Depression: A neurochemical threshold model of the relation between the illnesses. *Psychological Bulletin*, 1993; 113(1):23–43.

Martinsen, EW, Medhus, A, Sandvik, L. Effects of aerobic exercise on depression: a controlled Study, *Br Med J*, 1985; 291:109.

Nakajima, T. Amine precursor amino acid therapy: from neurochemical basis to clinical aspects. *Neurochem Res*, 1996; 21(2):251–58.

Venero, JL, Herrera, AJ, Machado, A, et al. Changes in neurotransmitter levels associated with the deficiency of some essential amino acids in the diet. *Br J Nutr*, 1992; 68(2):409–20.

Volz, HP, Kieser, M. Kava-kava extract: WS 1490 versus placebo in anxiety disorders—a randomized placebo-controlled 25-week outpatient trial. *Pharmacopsychiatry*, 1997; 30(1): 1–5.

Wells, AS, Read, NW, Laugharne, JD, et al. Alterations in mood after changing to a low-fat diet. *Br J Nutr*, 1998; 79(1):23–30.

Wyatt, KM. Efficacy of vitamin B_6 in the treatment of premenstrual syndrome: systematic review. *Br Med J*, 1999; 318(7195):1375–81.

OTHER BOOKS
AND RESOURCES

American Medical Association. *Essential Guide to Depression.* New York: Pocket Books, 1998.

Balch, JF, and Balch, PA. *Prescription for Nutritional Healing,* second edition. Garden City Park, NY: Avery Publishing Group, 1997.

Cass, H. *St. John's Wort: Nature's Blues Buster.* Garden City Park, NY: Avery Publishing Group, 1998.

Cass, H. *Kava: Nature's Answer to Stress, Anxiety, and Insomnia.* Rocklin, CA: Prima Publishing, 1998.

Clouatre, D. *All About SAM-e.* Garden City Park, NY: Avery Publishing Group, 1999.

Opler, LA. *Prozac and Other Psychiatric Drugs.* New York: Pocket Books, 1996.

Pauling, L. *How to Live Longer and Feel Better.* New York: W. H. Freeman and Company, 1986.

Reiter, RJ, and Robinson, J. *Melatonin: Your Body's Natural Wonder Drug.* New York: Bantam Books, 1995.

Sahelian, R. *5-HTP: Nature's Serotonin Solution.* Garden City Park, NY: Avery Publishing Group, 1998.

Slagle, P. *The Way Up from Down.* New York: Random House, 1987.

GreatLife Magazine
Consumer magazine with articles on vitamins, minerals, herbs, and foods.

Available for free at many health and natural food stores.

Let's Live Magazine
Consumer magazine with emphasis on the health benefits of vitamins, minerals, and herbs.

Customer service:
1-800-676-4333
P.O. Box 74908
Los Angeles, CA 90004

Subscriptions: 12 issues per year, $19.95 in the U.S.; $31.95 outside the U.S.

Physical Magazine
Magazine oriented to body builders and other serious athletes.

Customer service:
1-800-676-4333
P.O. Box 74908
Los Angeles, CA 90004

Subscriptions: 12 issues per year, $19.95 in the U.S.; $31.95 outside the U.S.

The Nutrition Reporter™ newsletter
Monthly newsletter that summarizes recent medical research on vitamins, minerals, and herbs.

Customer service:
P.O. Box 30246
Tucson, AZ 85751-0246
e-mail: jack@thenutritionreporter.com
www.nutritionreporter.com

Subscriptions: $26 per year (12 issues) in the U.S.; $32 U.S. or $48 CNC for Canada; $38 for other countries.

National Institute of Mental Health
Information Resources and Inquiries Branch
6001 Executive Boulevard
Bethesda, MD 20892-9663
301-443-4513
www.nimh.nih.gov

Depression and Related Affective Disorders Association (DRADA)
Meyer 3-181, 600 N. Wolfe Street
Baltimore, MD 21287-7381
410-955-4647
www.drada.org

American Psychological Association
750 First Street, N.E.
Washington, D.C. 20002-4242
800-374-2721
www.apa.org

Light Box Suppliers

The SunBox Company
19217 Orbit Drive
Gaithersberg, MD 20879
800-548-3968
www.sunbox.com

Apollo Light Systems, Inc.
376 S. Commerce Loop
Orem, UT 84058
800-545-9667
www.apollolight.com
e-mail: info@apollolight.com

INDEX